HOW TO CHOOSE THE RIGHT DOCTOR

7 things patients should look out for in health care Practitioners

Carmen M. Roberts

This book is designed to provide accurate and Authoritative information in regard to the subject matter covered. If expert assistance or counseling are needed, the service of a competent professional should be sought.

Table of Contents

Introduction

In the depths of a daunting health journey, I found myself caught in the labyrinth of medical consultations. My journey began with persistent symptoms that seemed to evade diagnosis. I navigated through various healthcare providers, each encounter laden with uncertainty.

I needed specialist care since I had a rare autoimmune illness. My illness was complicated by a multitude of symptoms, therefore I needed a doctor who was well-versed in the nuances of my disease. Finding the ideal healthcare provider, however, turned out to be a difficult process.

My journey began with well-intentioned general practitioners whose best attempts, despite their best efforts, were not enough to fully understand the intricacy of my condition. I had to put up with the aggravating results of generic treatments that barely touched the surface of my needs and incorrect diagnoses.

I ventured into the world of specialists, determined to locate the proper physician. I consulted specialists in neurology and rheumatology, among other specialties. However, I was unable to find a medical partner who was aware of the subtleties of my disease. The psychological toll of constant setbacks threatened to eclipse my optimism for a full recovery.

Amid a sea of medical appointments, I went into a support group for people facing comparable health issues. It was in this forum that I came across a ray of hope in the form of a fellow sufferer whose experience was strikingly similar to mine.

My unusual autoimmune illness was treated by a doctor I found thanks to this newfound connection. During the first meeting, I experienced a distinct sense of empathy, compassion, and a dedication to deciphering the intricate details of my health condition. This doctor cared about my health; he listened to me carefully and asked insightful questions.

The emotional load that had been on me for so long began to ease as my treatment plan came to pass. In addition to having the required medical training, the ideal physician understood the value of building a solid doctor-patient rapport.

My experience, which was characterized by tenacity and fortitude, served as the inspiration for my book, "How to Choose the Right Doctor." I emphasize in my poignant story the vital significance of having a health care professional who treats a patient's holistic requirements in addition to their illness. Echoing the central theme of my book, my story demonstrates the transformational power of collaborative and trusting cooperation between doctors and patients.

I encourage all patients who are struggling to understand the complexities of healthcare to look into the procedures described in the various chapters of this book which is not is not just a reference; but a road map that will enable you to make decisions that are best for your health. Gaining insight into these crucial factors will improve your chances of selecting the ideal healthcare partner and open the door to a more fulfilling and successful healthcare experience. I hope that the knowledge I've gained from this experience will give individuals starting their journey toward improved health a ray of hope.

Chapter 1

Understanding your Healthcare Needs

The path to the best possible healthcare starts with a deep awareness of oneself. This chapter argues that the first steps in selecting the best healthcare practitioner are self-awareness and reflection. You are invited to participate in a contemplative process that covers a range of factors related to your health and overall well-being before starting your search for a physician.

Evaluating Your Health Condition

You are asked to explore the details of your health situations in the area of self-reflection. What is your general health status and how does it affect your day-to-day activities? Think about things like your energy levels, sleep habits, and emotional health. Recognizing current illnesses and their effects on day-to-day functioning sets the stage for a more intelligent approach to medical care.

Identifying and recording symptoms is an essential part of this diagnostic process. What symptoms does your body show, and when does it show them? Knowing the frequency and intensity of your symptoms gives you important information to share with medical professionals, which can lead to a more precise diagnosis and individualized treatment plan.

Determining Your Particular Needs for Healthcare

As your general health becomes more apparent, the emphasis switches to determining your unique healthcare requirements. What are your long-term health objectives and what worries you right now? Setting priorities for your problems will help you find a healthcare professional with the necessary expertise more quickly.

Establishing health objectives is also very important. Whether your goals are pain relief, weight loss, or mental health, putting them into words will help you choose a physician whose qualifications match your desires. This proactive approach gives you the ability to take an active role in your healthcare process.

The Impact of Lifestyle Elements

Comprehending healthcare demands involves more than just symptoms; it also involves lifestyle decisions. What role do your sleep patterns, food, and level of activity play in your general well-being? Understanding how lifestyle factors are interrelated puts you in a better position to choose a physician who understands the holistic approach to health and can offer individualized advice.

The management of stress is an important factor. What is the effect of stress on your health and how do you manage it? For all-encompassing care, finding a physician who recognizes and treats health disorders related to stress is essential.

Building a Collaboration to Promote Holistic Health

Equipped with an all-encompassing comprehension of your well-being, this chapter urges you to view healthcare as a joint endeavor. It highlights how crucial it is to build a relationship with a healthcare professional who values your active participation in decision-making and who not only has the requisite medical skills. This cooperative strategy encourages a sense of shared accountability for reaching the best possible health results.

Managing Healthcare with Knowledge and assurance

The notion that self-awareness is essential for confidently and intelligently navigating the complicated world of healthcare is reaffirmed in the chapter's conclusion. You give yourself the capacity to advocate for your well-being and make educated decisions by actively participating in the process of identifying your healthcare needs. The acquired knowledge serves as a potent instrument for establishing a significant and fruitful collaboration with a healthcare practitioner, laying the groundwork for a path toward comprehensive well-being.

Chapter 2

Qualifications and Credentials

Finding the ideal physician to treat you is an exciting adventure in knowledge and skill. A patient's confidence in their selected practitioner is largely determined by their qualifications and credentials, which are the cornerstones of trust and assurance in the wide world of healthcare.

Dissecting the Expertise of Tapestry

The investigation starts with an engrossing trip through the training and credentials of a healthcare professional. Think of this procedure as similar to piecing together a tapestry, where each thread signifies a distinct learning and specialization milestone. A doctor's breadth of knowledge and dedication to their subject are demonstrated by interwoven medical degrees, residency training, and fellowship programs.

Board Certifications: The Ultimate Qualification

Examine the importance of board certificates, which are the most prestigious in the medical field. These credentials indicate that a physician has fulfilled the necessary coursework and training requirements as well as passed difficult exams to prove their expertise in a particular area of medicine. Understanding the significance of board certifications gives patients peace of mind that their preferred physician upholds higher standards of care and consistently pursues excellence in their specialty.

Licensing

Often overlooked in importance, licensing is the legal façade that validates a physician's right to practice medicine. Examine the subtleties of licensing as the essential component that guarantees patients that a provider is approved and recognized by the regulatory bodies that oversee medicine. This section clarifies how licensing functions as a safeguard, assuring patients that the person managing their health is, in fact, competent and permitted to do so.

Credentials in the Digital Age

It's critical to grasp how to navigate the digital world in the information era. This section of the chapter explains how patients can use Internet resources to confirm the credentials and training of a physician. This section gives patients the tools to investigate the qualifications of the doctor of their choosing on their own, using credible online directories and official medical board websites. It turns the seemingly difficult work into an interesting and approachable exploration voyage.

Adding Fun to Qualifications

Even though credentials and qualifications are a serious matter, this chapter adds a fun element to the story. It transforms the process of confirming a doctor's credentials into one of empowerment. You should view your healthcare as a ticket to a healthier life, and you take on the role of watchful protector of your health by carefully examining a doctor's credentials. This section encourages patients to see obtaining qualifications as an exciting and dynamic way to learn about the fields of knowledge that will impact their healthcare experience, rather than as a tedious and bureaucratic process.

To sum up, this chapter exudes the thrill of exploration. It makes clear how to locate a physician whose credentials match the caliber of care you should receive. As you read this chapter, picture yourself as an explorer traveling a field of expertise, with the knowledge to identify the credentials and qualifications that will lead to a reliable and competent healthcare collaboration.

Chapter 3

Experience and Expertise

One cannot stress the importance of a doctor's experience and knowledge in the ever-changing field of healthcare. This chapter explores the important aspects that seasoned experience and specialized expertise bring to the forefront of the patient-doctor relationship as patients set out on their search to select the ideal healthcare provider.

Getting Around in the Years of Practice

Experience is the development of knowledge and skill as well as the passing of time. I can attest to the effect that years of experience in the field can have on the standard of care because of my personal experience as a patient and medical professional. An experienced practitioner can negotiate issues with a seasoned perspective because they frequently have a lot of knowledge gathered from a variety of patient circumstances. To feel confident and assured about their medical advice, patients are urged to think about the advantages of selecting a physician whose experience matches their unique healthcare needs.

Particularized Fields of Knowledge

My own experience emphasizes how crucial a doctor's skill is, particularly in terms of specialization. A physician's knowledge base is not limited to general practice; it frequently spreads to specialized fields. The need to find a healthcare professional whose experience matches the patient's particular health issues is discussed in this section. As a patient, I was reassured by experts whose knowledge aligned with my particular health issues, guaranteeing a more accurate and customized approach to treatment. Expertise demonstrates a profound dedication to a certain area, enabling medical professionals to refine their abilities and remain up to date with the most recent developments.

The Changing Confluence of Innovation and Experience

Experience and invention are intertwined; they do not exist in isolation. I've learned the value of this dynamic intersection from my personal experience as a patient and healthcare advocate. A physician's ability to incorporate cutting-edge technologies and treatment modalities with well-established procedures results in a dynamic medical setting. Patients are advised to look for healthcare professionals who have an innovative outlook and create a setting where conventional wisdom and state-of-the-art approaches coexist. This dynamic approach, which demonstrates the power of experience mixed with innovation, has, in my view, been a driver for better health results.

The Center of Expertise in the Patient-Centered Approach

A patient-centered approach reveals the genuine value of experience and competence. Having experienced both ends of the healthcare system, I understand how crucial it is for physicians to place a high priority on individualized care. In addition to their medical expertise, a skilled and knowledgeable healthcare provider also possesses empathy and a sympathetic awareness of the individual requirements of each patient. This patient-centric approach guarantees that healthcare is a collaborative process where the doctor's expertise is customized to the patient's unique health narrative, rather than a one-size-fits-all undertaking. Throughout my journey, I have seen firsthand how a patient-centered approach can truly revolutionize healthcare and emphasize the core principles of true medical knowledge.

This chapter, on its whole, presents a clear picture of the mutually beneficial relationship that exists between experience and competence. It provides a thorough understanding of the subtle advantages of selecting a physician with a wealth of expertise, a particular focus, and a dedication to a patient-centered approach by guiding patients via personal tales and expert insights. Understanding and valuing these attributes becomes essential for people navigating the healthcare system to have a meaningful and productive relationship with a healthcare practitioner who supports their individual health goals.

Chapter 4

Communication Skills

Effective communication between a doctor and patient is essential to a successful medical journey in the complex dance of healthcare. It is more than just a conversation. This chapter explains the critical role that communication skills play in the doctor-patient interaction and highlights why choosing the correct healthcare provider depends on having effective communication skills.

The Art of Connection

Doctors who can fully comprehend their patients' voices are masters of the art of connection, which is the foundation of communication. The expert communication skills of a physician act as a compass for patients as they discuss symptoms, worries, and medical history, leading them through the diagnostic process. I've seen from my personal experiences how much of an impact a doctor's capacity for active listening and empathy-building can have on the patient experience as a whole. This section goes into the value of doctors who not only hear but genuinely listen to their patients, generating a sense of understanding and partnership.

Deciphering Medical Jargon

Understanding the complexities of healthcare frequently requires navigating a maze of medical jargon. In this situation, the doctor's ability to simplify difficult ideas into easily understood information is what constitutes effective communication. Looking back on my path, I've seen that doctors who communicate not only provide patients with the knowledge to empower them but also foster an atmosphere of openness and trust. This section of the chapter delves into the significance of physicians who are adept at demystifying medical information so that patients can actively participate in their treatment decisions.

Empathy in Action

The link between medical knowledge and human comprehension is empathy. The significant influence of physicians who exhibit empathy in their work is explained in this section. I know from my own experiences as a patient the therapeutic value of a physician who understands the psychological and emotional components of illness in addition to diagnosing and prescribing. Genuine care from a doctor cultivates a therapeutic alliance and provides a comfortable environment in which patients can talk candidly about their health issues.

Building Communication to Foster Trust

Any meaningful relationship between a patient and a doctor is built on trust, and trust is developed via effective communication. In this section of the chapter, the subtleties of communication that foster trust are examined through the lens of both personal and professional experiences. It highlights how a strong foundation of trust may be built on a doctor's openness, honesty, and willingness to participate in honest communication. A collaborative collaboration between the patient and the doctor is formed through excellent communication, which covers everything from treatment options to addressing concerns.

Managing Cultural Sensitivities

Effective communication in the diverse field of healthcare includes recognizing and managing cultural sensitivities. This section emphasizes how important it is for medical professionals to embrace cultural competence and acknowledge the distinct needs and viewpoints of patients from different origins. As I think back on my experiences, I've learned to value medical professionals who actively attempt to comprehend and include diversity in their communication strategies in addition to showing respect for it.

Making Use of Technology

The digital era has expanded communication beyond in-person meetings. The use of technology as a vital instrument for healthcare communication is examined in this section of the chapter. Through the use of encrypted messaging platforms and telemedicine sessions, technology is used to improve accessibility and encourage ongoing communication between the patient and the physician. Based on my own experiences, technology can significantly enhance the patient experience and maintain communication as a continuous and dynamic process.

Finally, this chapter reveals the many facets of communication skills as the foundation of the patient-physician interaction. It provides a thorough understanding of the revolutionary effect that good communication can have on the patient experience. The chapter highlights the importance of communication skills in selecting the best healthcare provider and sheds light on their many facets, from the art of connection to technology use.

Chapter 5

Patient Reviews and Recommendations

Patients have access to a valuable resource in the digital age while searching for the best healthcare provider: the opinions and experiences of other patients. This chapter explores the value of patient reviews and recommendations, showing how they can drastically alter the decision-making process and how they play a part in the author's quest to identify the best medical option.

Getting Around the Patient Review Landscape

Patient reviews serve as a compass in the wide terrain of healthcare choices. This section looks at the various ways that patients communicate their experiences, from word-of-mouth referrals to internet platforms. Based on my quest for a medical collaborator, I found that patient reviews include a plethora of information. It became an indispensable component of my decision-making process, offering insightful information on the dynamics between patients and doctors, the efficacy of treatments, and the general pleasure of people who had gone through the healthcare system before me.

Gaining Knowledge from Other Patients

In contrast to the clinical descriptions that are frequently found in medical literature, patient reviews provide an actual voice of experience. When I thought back on my own experience, I found comfort and direction in the stories of people who had experienced comparable medical difficulties. Their experiences turned into sources of inspiration and useful insight, providing a more nuanced understanding of the characteristics of healthcare professionals. This section explores the value of shared experiences, highlighting the distinctive perspectives that patients can offer to supplement more conventional sources of knowledge.

My Individual Exploration Through Patient Testimonials

In a coincidental turn of events, patient reviews were essential to my own medical experience. It was from the sincere testimonies of people who had experienced a similar problem to mine that I found a physician whose knowledge and patient-centered approach stood out. Patient evaluations led me to a healthcare provider who would later be essential in my recovery, bridging the gap between my uncertainty and a possible answer.

Handling the Variations in Reviews

Star ratings provide an overview of overall satisfaction, but this section explores the subtleties of patient reviews in more detail. It invites readers to delve further into the in-depth narratives and look behind the numerical numbers. Patients can match their preferences with a healthcare provider's attributes by knowing the specifics included in reviews, which cover anything from communication methods to bedside manners. This refined method guarantees a deeper comprehension of a physician's areas of strength and possible growth.

Word-of-mouth Advice: A Well-Traveled Custom

Word-of-mouth recommendations are still a tried-and-true method in healthcare decision-making, in addition to internet platforms. The importance of referrals from friends, family, and coworkers is discussed in this section. These first-hand accounts have particular significance since they frequently demonstrate the rapport and confidence that patients have developed with their medical professionals. Looking back on my own experience, I realized that the way I first discovered the doctor who would play a key role in my medical narrative was via a word-of-mouth recommendation.

Differentiating Sincere Evaluations

This chapter acknowledges skepticism while simultaneously providing insightful patient reviews. It instructs readers on how to separate objective assessments from possible biases and emphasizes the value of analyzing the general tone and reoccurring themes rather than depending just on individual remarks. With this sophisticated approach, patients are guaranteed to be able to make well-informed decisions based on a fair assessment of the advantages and disadvantages of a healthcare provider.

This thorough chapter concludes by elucidating the complex function that patient testimonials and recommendations play in the process of choosing a physician. The transforming power of shared experiences is shown throughout the chapter, from online platforms to personal recommendations. It emphasizes how important a role patient reviews had in the author's journey and provides evidence of the insightful information that can help people choose the best healthcare provider for their particular circumstances.

Chapter 6

Office Atmosphere and Staff

The environment of a doctor's office and the mannerisms of the support personnel are crucial factors in determining the whole patient experience in the complex field of healthcare. In this chapter, the importance of staff dynamics and office atmosphere is discussed, along with how they affect patients' overall satisfaction with healthcare services and their general well-being.

The Entry: A Comforting or Uncomfortable Preface

The experience of visiting a doctor's office frequently starts at the door, and the ambiance created there determines the overall mood of the appointment. This section examines the understated yet significant components that add to the overall atmosphere. The entrance becomes the first step toward either comfort or worry, depending on how well-kept the waiting space is and how friendly the welcome is. Based on my personal experiences, I've learned to value the ability of a friendly environment to allay fears and encourage optimism.

Beyond the Chairs and Magazines in the Waiting Area

The waiting area represents the doctor's dedication to the comfort of his or her patients and is more than just a room with chairs and periodicals. This section of the chapter explores the subtleties of a thoughtfully planned waiting area, stressing the value of creating a tranquil space. A well-designed environment can enhance a patient's overall well-being by creating an environment that is favorable to candid dialogue and the development of trust.

Staff Interactions

One of the most important aspects of the office environment is the interactions between the supporting staff and patients. The importance of staff interactions as the personal touch that improves the patient experience is discussed in this section. Their professionalism, sensitivity, and approachability, from receptionists to nurses, add

31

to a caring environment. My personal experiences have demonstrated the transforming power of a staff that is empathetic and supportive, fostering an atmosphere where patients feel respected and cherished.

Organization and Efficiency

The organization and efficiency of a doctor's office are indicators of high-quality care, not just practical considerations. This section of the chapter explores the significance of efficient procedures, on-time arrival, and clear communication. A well-organized office not only improves the experience for patients but also shows that the staff is dedicated to providing careful, comprehensive care.

The Impact of Workplace Culture on General Healthcare

Even though every patient has unique health problems, a doctor's office environment is universally significant. This part broadens the focus to investigate how a friendly and well-organized setting affects the general impression of the quality of healthcare. A friendly environment in the workplace can accommodate a variety of healthcare requirements, from regular check-ups to more complicated medical problems.

Beyond the Consultation Room

The consultation room is just one place where the supporting staff's professionalism shines through; it affects the patient's whole healthcare experience. This chapter challenges readers to think about how office culture and staff relationships may affect their level of satisfaction with healthcare services in general. A patient's assessment of the total quality of treatment is influenced by the support they receive from the time of admission until their interactions after the consultation.

Creating a Healing Environment

This thorough chapter concludes by highlighting the critical impact that staff dynamics and office atmosphere have on the healthcare experience of patients. It highlights how crucial it is to create a healing space that encompasses not just medical knowledge but also the general atmosphere of the doctor's office. The chapter encourages readers to acknowledge the significant influence that a well-designed environment may have on their well-being, from the first entrance to contacts with personnel, thereby contributing to a happy and comprehensive healthcare journey.

Chapter 7

Accessibility and Availability

These factors have become crucial cornerstones in the pursuit of high-quality healthcare that profoundly impacts the patient experience. This chapter explores the critical role these ideas play, highlighting their influence on healthcare outcomes and narrating how they improved the author's health journey.

The Fundamentals of Accessibility

The ease with which patients can access and interact with healthcare services is included in the concept of accessibility. This section addresses the necessity of breaking down barriers to access, ensuring that healthcare is within reach for persons from all walks of life. Looking back on my health journey, I can attest to the fact that timely treatments made possible by easily accessible healthcare can prevent health conditions from getting worse and promote overall well-being.

Geographical Proximity

The accessibility of healthcare services is significantly influenced by their geographic closeness. This section of the chapter examines how a patient's capacity to seek prompt medical attention may be impacted by a doctor's office location. According to my observations, having a medical professional nearby not only made things more convenient but also promoted routine checkups and preventive health care. The proximity of a medical facility serves as a trigger for timely medical intervention.

Availability of Appointments

A patient's ability to receive timely care is influenced by the delicate balance of appointment availability. The significance of a healthcare provider's dedication to providing accessible appointment times is explored in this section. Looking back on my personal experience, I've concluded that having appointments available for both routine check-ups and urgent issues helped to provide a sense of security. Patients can handle their healthcare demands without needless delays because of its accessibility.

Telemedicine and Flexible Hours

Healthcare accessibility has changed in the current day to include telemedicine choices and flexible hours. This section of the chapter examines how these modifications have a transformative effect. In light of my experiences, I value the flexibility that works with different schedules and enables people to put their health first without sacrificing other obligations. In particular, telemedicine has become a bridge to healthcare services from the comfort of one's home, making it a revolutionary feature of accessibility.

Benefits of this Factor on my Health Journey

During the course of my health journey, availability and accessibility have been revolutionary. Regular check-ups and prompt interventions were made easier by having a healthcare practitioner within reasonable travel distance and by providing flexible appointment times. I was able to get medical advice without being constrained by schedules or geographical distances thanks to the availability of telemedicine solutions. All of these factors helped me take a proactive and preventive attitude to my health, which improved my general well-being.

Reducing Healthcare Inequalities

This chapter recognizes the systemic effects of increased accessibility in healthcare, going beyond personal experiences. It becomes our joint duty to address gaps in healthcare service access. A dedication to improving accessibility means that people may receive the care they require, no matter what their circumstances or background may be. This leads to a more fair healthcare environment.

An Opening to the Best Medical Care

To sum up, availability and accessibility serve as doors to the best healthcare. This thorough chapter emphasizes how crucial a role they play in molding the patient's experience and improving health outcomes. A proactive and patient-centric approach to healthcare is sparked by the ideas of accessibility and availability, which transcend geographic boundaries and encourage the adoption of contemporary healthcare conveniences. The chapter urges readers to take these factors into account when making healthcare decisions, realizing how transformative they can be in creating a pleasant and easy-to-access healthcare experience.

Chapter 8

Insurance and Payment Options

The practical factors of insurance coverage and payment options stand out as crucial elements in the complex web of healthcare considerations that have a substantial impact on patients' overall health. This chapter discusses the value of having a variety of payment alternatives and comprehending insurance coverage, highlighting their part in guaranteeing that everyone has access to inexpensive healthcare.

The Insurance Assurance: Protecting Health and Assets

Insurance acts as a barrier, preserving patients' financial security as well as their health. The several advantages of having comprehensive insurance coverage are examined in this section. I've learned to value the assurance that comes with knowing that medical costs are paid for after giving some thought to my personal healthcare experiences. Insurance is a safety net that creates a sense of confidence and enables people to prioritize their health without constantly worrying about financial obligations, from routine check-ups to unanticipated medical emergencies.

Getting Around Insurance Policies

Gaining an understanding of insurance coverage can be a challenging but rewarding process. The significance of patients actively utilizing their insurance coverage is covered in detail in this section of the chapter. Making educated healthcare decisions is made possible by having a thorough understanding of all the elements of coverage, including co-payments and deductibles. Patients are better able to take advantage of their benefits when they have a clear understanding of insurance coverage, which encourages timely treatments as well as preventive care.

Payment Options Function

The link between healthcare services and financial viability is payment alternatives. This section examines the wide variety of payment alternatives and how important they are in promoting affordability and accessibility. When I think back on my personal experiences, I've discovered that accepting different forms of payment or providing flexible payment plans are two ways that healthcare providers can foster an inclusive healthcare atmosphere. This flexibility guarantees that people can receive the treatment they require, irrespective of their financial situation.

Healthcare Delay Prevention

Having access to timely healthcare should never be impeded by financial concerns. This section of the chapter focuses on the ways that flexible payment plans and insurance coverage help to avoid delays in getting medical care. People with accessible payment alternatives are more likely to seek care promptly, limiting the escalation of health issues and promoting a proactive culture of health management. This includes routine screenings and treating minor health concerns.

The Benefits of Positive Ripples for Public Health

Comprehensive insurance and adjustable payment plans have a good knock-on effect that improves public health in addition to individual health results. This section examines how lowering healthcare costs benefits a stronger, healthier community. Affordable healthcare access encourages people to prioritize preventative care, which lessens the overall strain on the healthcare system and fosters a shared commitment to well-being.

A Comprehensive Strategy for Healthcare Accessibility

This chapter concludes by emphasizing the comprehensive approach to healthcare accessibility that is made possible by extensive insurance coverage and adjustable payment plans. It highlights how financial concerns and health results are mutually reinforcing. This method helps create a better society where everyone can actively participate in their well-being by promoting a healthcare system that everyone can use without financial limitations. The chapter promotes a proactive approach to financial and health-related decision-making by encouraging readers to investigate and comprehend their insurance alternatives.

Chapter 9

Building a Trusted Patient-Doctor Relationship

A reliable doctor-patient relationship is the cornerstone of efficient healthcare. To emphasize the transformational power of a true partnership in healthcare, this final chapter navigates the fundamental relevance of creating a connection based on trust, demonstrating its clear correlation with the previously described criteria and incorporating the author's narrative.

The Basis of Trust

It becomes clear as we go through the fundamental requirements covered in previous chapters—insurance, accessibility, office atmosphere, patient reviews, experience, qualifications, and communication skills—that each requirement adds to the base upon which trust is constructed. Each component of a trustworthy doctor-patient connection—from the physician's experience to the friendly environment of the office, from open communication to the guarantee of easily accessible and reasonably priced healthcare—intertwines to build the foundation of that relationship.

The Symphonic Link

Consider the requirements as individual notes in a musical composition, each contributing to the overall harmony of healthcare. Qualifications and experience create the tone, communication skills choreograph the discourse, patient reviews provide a chorus of shared experiences, the office setting becomes the backdrop, and accessibility plays the melody of convenience, and insurance acts as the reassuring rhythm. The soul-stirring tune that unites everything in this symphony of collaborative care is the trust between the physician and the patient.

A Testament to Trust's Transformative Power

The importance of a trustworthy doctor-patient connection became abundantly clear to me during my journey. In addition to medical knowledge, navigating health issues requires a partnership based on mutual respect and understanding. The standards described in this book were more than just check boxes; they were essential tools in helping patients and healthcare providers develop a trusting relationship.

The doctor's training and expertise gave people confidence, and his ability to communicate well fostered a feeling of group decision-making. Patient testimonials offered perceptions of other people's experiences, strengthening the feeling of camaraderie throughout the medical process. An environment free from stress was guaranteed by accessible options and a friendly office attitude. Financial obstacles were eliminated by the variety of payment methods and extensive insurance coverage, enabling an emphasis on health rather than concerns over expenses.

As I navigated the trip, it became clear that the doctor-patient relationship—one based on open communication, trust, and a shared commitment to well-being—is the fundamental component of healthcare.

Building Trust for the Best Results in Healthcare

Not only is a trustworthy doctor-patient connection a positive feature of healthcare, but it also has a direct impact on results. This section looks at how trust can lead to higher patient engagement, better adherence to treatment programs, and overall health improvements. Patients' open communication, conscientious adherence to medical recommendations, and active participation in their care are all increased when they have confidence in their healthcare providers, which ultimately leads to improved patient outcomes.

Companionship: The Foundation of Faith

Mutual respect is the cornerstone of a trustworthy doctor-patient relationship. This section of the chapter highlights how trust is a reciprocal relationship and how both sides may contribute to its growth. Physicians who actively involve their patients in decision-making and value their opinions create a trusting atmosphere. In a similar vein, patients who value their physicians' knowledge and adhere to their advice foster cooperative relationships that improve patient outcomes.

The Vital Essence of healthcare

To sum up, developing a trustworthy doctor-patient relationship becomes the most important aspect of healthcare. This chapter integrates the criteria covered in the book, showing how each component contributes differently to the development of trust. The author's narrative demonstrates the transforming potential of a trust-based relationship, where healthcare is transformed into a cooperative journey toward well-being. This chapter urges readers to prioritize and actively participate in the formation of a trustworthy doctor-patient relationship as they begin their healthcare decisions. This relationship should go beyond simple medical transactions and instead become a shared commitment to health and healing.

Conclusion

As we come to the end of this investigation into the nuances of selecting the ideal physician, it is appropriate to consider the transforming potential contained within these pages. Your trip through the requirements—experience, education, patient testimonials, office environment, ease of access, insurance, and the epitome of a reliable doctor-patient relationship—has served as a compass to help you make knowledgeable and empowered healthcare decisions.

My health story, in the tradition of personal narratives, is a source of inspiration, perseverance, and hope. By diligently adhering to the aforementioned standards, my health has not only stabilized but has improved. To successfully navigate health difficulties, a partnership based on trust, excellent communication, and a supportive environment has been essential.

But as this book comes to an end, one more word of caution is necessary. Finding the correct doctor is a complex process, and although this book offers a clear route, you must proceed with caution. Healthcare decisions have significant ramifications, and each person's journey is specially molded by their circumstances, preferences, and health requirements.

It is advised that you approach the selection procedure with diligence and actively participate in the given criteria. When starting your healthcare journey, think about the credentials, explore experiences, value clear communication, assess patient feedback, evaluate the office environment, place a high value on accessibility, comprehend your insurance options, and, most importantly, cultivate a trustworthy relationship with your healthcare provider.

My experience serves as a reminder that achieving optimal health requires teamwork in addition to being an inspiration. A good physician is more than just a medicine specialist; they are a collaborator, mentor, and advocate on your path to wellness.

This conclusion, in the spirit of empowerment, invites you to take charge of your health, be proactive in selecting the appropriate physician, and see the given criteria as dynamic components that work together to create a rewarding and successful healthcare partnership rather than as inflexible checklists.

I hope that your path to better health is marked by wise decisions, enduring connections, and a dedication to well-being. Here's to navigating the intricacies of healthcare with resilience, knowledge, and the conviction that the appropriate doctor is a critical ally in the goal of a healthier and happier life.